LOSE 30LBS IN 30 DAYS

1200
CALORIE DIET FOR
FAST WEIGHT-LOSS

DIET GUIDE COOKBOOK

Ultimate Low carb high protein meal plan with recipes for fat loss, high energy and to stay shredded

Brittany Rice

TABLE OF CONTENT

DO YOU PROMISE ?

Are you tired of feeling trapped in a body that doesn't reflect the vibrant person inside? Imagine shedding those extra pounds and emerging as the confident, energetic, and unstoppable version of yourself. It's time to break free from the weight that's been holding you back.

You deserve to feel incredible every single day. *But right now, excess weight might be clouding your brilliance, preventing you from seizing life's opportunities. Don't let it stand in your way any longer!*

Picture this: A life where you wake up invigorated, excited to take on the day with boundless energy. Imagine the freedom of effortlessly fitting into your favorite clothes, feeling comfortable and confident in your own skin.

Weight loss isn't just about numbers on a scale—it's reclaiming your narrative, your self-worth, and your happiness. It's about becoming the best version of yourself, both physically and mentally.

You have dreams to chase, goals to achieve, and experiences waiting for you. But sometimes, excess weight can become a barrier, limiting your potential and dimming your shine. Let go of the weight that's been holding you back and step into a future where nothing can stop you.

Join countless others on this transformative journey towards health, confidence, and self-empowerment. You have the power to sculpt your destiny and create the life you've always envisioned.

It's time to take charge. Embrace the challenge. Choose yourself and commit to unleashing your true potential. The path to a brighter, more vibrant you begins now.

INTRODUCTION

WELCOME MESSAGE

We are aware that starting a weight loss journey may be an exciting and intimidating experience. But do not worry, this cookbook will make the trip a tasty and exciting one. It's intended to transform your perspective on eating as well as assist you in losing weight.

You'll discover an abundance of delicious dishes designed to entice your taste buds and help you achieve your weight loss goals in these pages. Every meal, which ranges from delicious breakfasts to filling dinners and delectable snacks in between, has been carefully chosen to achieve the ideal ratio of flavor to nutrition.

This is a roadmap guiding you towards healthier eating habits and a lifestyle that fuels your body and soul. You'll discover tips, tricks, and insights that will empower you to make mindful food choices and embrace a more vibrant, energized life.

Recall that the goal here is to nourish your body with scrumptious, healthful meals that will leave you feeling full and energized, not about restriction or strict guidelines. It's about enjoying each bite as you move closer to your health objectives.

So take a deep breath, explore, and allow these recipes to serve as the foundation for your metamorphosis. Accept this trip with open arms and a desire to experience the amazing flavors that eating a healthy diet has to offer.

So, dive in, explore, and let these recipes become the building blocks of your transformation. Embrace this journey with an open heart and a zest for discovering the incredible flavors that healthful eating has to offer.

HOW TO USE THIS COOKBOOK

1. Introduction:

- Begin by reading the Introduction to familiarize yourself with the cookbook's purpose and structure.

- Understand the importance of the 1200-calorie diet and how it can contribute to your weight-loss goals.

2. Getting Started:

- Evaluate your weight-loss goals and learn how to mentally and physically prepare for this journey.

- Refer to the Essential Shopping List to ensure you have the necessary ingredients for success.

3. 1200-Calorie Diet Basics:

- Explore the fundamentals of the 1200-calorie diet, including insights into macronutrients and tips for creating balanced meals.

- Discover effective portion control techniques to optimize your calorie intake.

4. High Protein Recipes:

- Find a variety of breakfast, lunch, dinner, and snack recipes rich in protein to support your weight-loss journey.

5. Low Carb Wonders:

- Learn about carb substitutes and alternatives that fit into the low-carb philosophy.

- Explore recipes that minimize carbohydrate intake while maintaining delicious flavors.

6. High Fiber Delicacies:

- Understand the significance of fiber in weight loss and explore recipes that are both delicious and fiber-rich.

- Discover creative snack ideas packed with essential dietary fiber.

7. Meal Planning and Sample Menus:

- Utilize the provided weekly meal plans and daily sample menus to streamline your dietary choices.

- Gain valuable tips for successful meal planning and execution.

8. Exercise and Lifestyle Support:

- Learn how to incorporate exercise routines into your weight-loss journey.

- Discover healthy lifestyle tips to complement your dietary efforts.

9. Tracking Progress:

Examine strategies for tracking your efforts toward weight loss and marking accomplishments.

- Seek advice on how to modify the strategy to suit your changing requirements.

10. FAQs and Troubleshooting:

- Find solutions to common problems and answers to frequently asked issues.

- Acquire tactics for surmounting obstacles and managing downturns.

11. Conclusion:

- Take in these parting words of wisdom as you get ready to start this life-changing adventure.

- Think of the cookbook as a tool to help you maintain your healthy lifestyle after the first thirty days.

12. Appendix:

To quickly define concepts, consult the glossary.

Make easy work of finding your favorite recipes with the recipe index.

- Look into more resources for inspiration and help in the future.

We invite you to use this cookbook as a thorough guide to help you reach your weight-loss objectives while encouraging a balanced, healthful lifestyle. Keep in mind that every voyage is different, so feel free to alter the schedules and recipes to fit your requirements. I hope your journey to a better, happier version of yourself goes well!

UNDERSTANDING THE 1200-CALORIE DIET

Why is the 1200-calorie diet the main focus of this cookbook, and what does it entail? Essentially, this strategy is a planned diet that centers around consuming approximately 1200 calories daily. It's important to remember that everyone has different calorie requirements depending on their age, gender, weight, degree of exercise, and general health. Although it's a starting point, the 1,200 calorie threshold is not a universally applicable answer.

This cookbook is about making every calorie matter, not just cutting back on calories. It's a thorough manual full of delectable recipes that have been painstakingly created to make sure you get the maximum nutrition and enjoyment out of every meal.

The genius of this strategy lies in the fact that it aims to transform your connection with food rather than merely reducing caloric intake. It's about eating full, nutrient-dense foods that help your weight loss objectives while also nourishing your body.

Within the constraints of a calorie-conscious approach, the dishes included within these pages are more than just meals; they're a celebration of tastes, textures, and inventiveness. Every meal, which ranges from fulfilling evenings to fiber-rich lunches and high-protein breakfasts, is designed to optimize flavor and nutrition while controlling your caloric intake.

However, keep in mind that a 1200 calorie diet is neither a short-term or magic cure. It's a chance to set off on a path toward portion control, mindful eating, and healthier eating habits. It's about laying the groundwork for a way of living that will sustain your health over time. We wish you well on your trip, and hope you approach it with curiosity, resolve, and self-compassion. Remember that the objective is not just to reduce weight but to become a healthier, more positive version of yourself.

So explore these pages, try out the recipes, and feast your eyes on the possibilities. Together, let's explore the amazing possibilities of the 1200 calorie diet and set out on a life-changing journey to a happier, healthier version of ourselves.

CHAPTER 1: GETTING STARTED

ASSESSING YOUR WEIGHT-LOSS GOALS

1. **Reflect on Your Why:** Start by asking yourself why you are starting this weight-loss journey. Is it to improve your well-being, get back your self-esteem, or just feel better about yourself? The key to your success is knowing why you do what you do.

2. **Define Your Goals:** Establish SMART goals—specific, measurable, achievable, relevant, and time-bound. Clearly define success for you, whether it's losing a specific amount of weight, getting into a certain size clothes, or improving health markers.

3. **Consider Realistic Expectations:** As important as enthusiasm is, reasonable expectations must also be set. Healthy weight loss usually involves losing 1-2 pounds every week, so instead of concentrating only on quick fixes, have patience and enjoy the ride.

4. **Account for Health Factors:** Consider the potential impact of any dietary restrictions, physical constraints, or underlying health concerns on your weight-loss journey. Speaking with a nutritionist or medical expert

might offer insightful advice specific to your requirements.

5. Measure Progress Beyond the Scale: Losing weight is about more than just the weight on the scale. Tracking additional success metrics like higher energy, better sleep, more stamina, or fit in clothes should be taken into consideration. These small triumphs can provide a great deal of motivation.

6. Create Milestones: Divide your long-term objective into more manageable, shorter deadlines. Celebrate these accomplishments since they demonstrate your growth and your dedication to your health and wellbeing.

PREPARING MENTALLY AND PHYSICALLY

Take a minute to emotionally and physically ready yourself for the amazing adventure ahead before plunging into the delectable dishes and meal plans included in this cookbook.

Mindset Matters: The mind is where success starts. Adopt an optimistic outlook and concentrate on the advantages of leading a healthier lifestyle. Have faith in your capacity to transform your life, and resolve to treat yourself with kindness while you go through this process. Keep in mind that your goal is to improve your well-being, not only lose weight.

Set Realistic Goals: Make sure your goals are realistic and well-defined. Divide them into more manageable benchmarks that you can acknowledge as you go. Setting realistic goals helps to avoid overwhelming emotions and paves the way for long-term growth.

Educate Yourself: You have the most power when you know. Recognize the underlying ideas of the 1200 calorie, high-protein, low-carb, high-fiber diet that you are about to start. Find out how nutrient-rich foods and portion sizes affect your overall health and ability to lose weight.

Clear Your Space: Set up your environment and kitchen for success. Get rid of any unhealthy, enticing items from your fridge and pantry. Ensure that you have enough of the ingredients listed in this cookbook so that you can prepare healthy meals.

Build Support Systems: Talk about your experience with loved ones, friends, or a support group. During trying times, having a solid support network can offer accountability, inspiration, and encouragement.

Prioritize Self-Care: It's just as crucial to focus on your mental and emotional well-being as it is on your physical health. Choose leisure pursuits that make you happy and content, such as hiking, writing in a diary, or meditation. Take care of yourself on all levels.

Physical Readiness: See a healthcare provider before beginning any new workout or diet program. To ensure a safe and successful trip, make sure you're physically prepared for this excursion and heed their instructions.

ESSENTIAL SHOPPING LIST

To help you stock your pantry and refrigerator with the necessities for your life-changing culinary journey, we've put up an essential shopping list.

Proteins:
- Skinless chicken breast
- Turkey breast
- Lean cuts of beef or pork
- Fish (such as salmon, tuna, or cod)
- Eggs and egg whites
- Greek yogurt or low-fat dairy options
- Plant-based proteins like tofu or tempeh

Vegetables:

- Leafy greens (spinach, kale, lettuce)

- Cruciferous veggies (broccoli, cauliflower)

- Bell peppers

- Zucchini

- Asparagus

- Mushrooms

- Tomatoes

Fruits:

- Berries (strawberries, blueberries, raspberries)

- Apples

- Citrus fruits (lemons, oranges)

- Avocado

Whole Grains and Legumes:

- Quinoa

- Brown rice

- Lentils

- Chickpeas

- Whole-grain bread or wraps

Nuts and Seeds:

- Almonds

- Walnuts

- Chia seeds

- Flaxseeds

Dairy/Dairy Substitutes:

- Unsweetened almond milk or other non-dairy alternatives

- Low-fat cheese options (if desired)

- Cottage cheese (low-fat or fat-free)

Condiments and Flavorings:

- Olive oil or avocado oil

- Herbs and spices (oregano, basil, cumin, turmeric)

- Low-sodium soy sauce or tamari

- Mustard

- Vinegar (balsamic, apple cider)

- Hot sauce

Miscellaneous:

- Unsweetened cocoa powder

- Stevia or another preferred low-calorie sweetener

- Herbal teas

Remember, this list forms the foundation for crafting nutrient-packed meals designed to support your weight-loss goals while keeping you satisfied and energized.

CHAPTER 2 : 1200-CALORIE DIET BASICS

UNDERSTANDING MACRONUTRIENTS

Starting a diet with 1,200 calories provides a path toward a well-balanced diet. Carbs, proteins, and fats are the macronutrients that are the foundation of this dietary journey.

1. **Carbohydrates:** Your body uses them as its main energy source to power your daily activities. Choose complex carbs over simple sugars in a diet of 1,200 calories or less, such as whole grains, legumes, and vegetables. These complex carbohydrates provide long-lasting energy that helps you avoid energy crashes and feel fuller for longer.

2. **Proteins:** Vital for muscle repair and growth, proteins are a crucial component of your diet. Aim for lean sources such as poultry, fish, tofu, legumes, and low-fat dairy to maximize protein intake while keeping calorie counts in check. Protein also aids in satiety, helping you feel satisfied and reducing cravings.

3. **Fats:** Despite their often-maligned reputation, healthy fats are essential for various bodily functions. Opt for sources like avocados, nuts, seeds, and olive oil to

incorporate healthy fats into your 1200-calorie diet. These fats support heart health, aid in nutrient absorption, and contribute to feeling full and satisfied.

It's important to balance these macronutrients within a 1200 calorie framework in order to meet your daily energy and satisfaction needs as well as your nutritional needs. Every macronutrient has a distinct effect on your general health, and a well-balanced diet plan will make the most of these benefits.

Recall that although monitoring macronutrients is crucial, quality is just as significant as quantity. Choose complete, nutrient-dense foods that are high in important vitamins, minerals, and antioxidants in addition to calories.

This cookbook's recipes and meal planning are built upon our understanding of macronutrients. With a focus on your general health and well-being, we want to help you achieve your weight loss objectives by utilizing the power of balanced nutrition within a 1200 calorie framework.

CREATING BALANCED MEALS

The three main macronutrients of a well-balanced 1,200-calorie meal are carbs, proteins, and fats. Each is essential for supplying energy and maintaining biological processes.

- Proteins: Try to get your protein from lean foods like fish, poultry, tofu, or lentils. Proteins maintain your feeling of fullness, help repair damaged muscles, and help control blood sugar levels.

- Carbs: Choose complex carbohydrates from fruits, vegetables, and whole grains. They offer long-lasting energy as well as vital elements including fiber, vitamins, and minerals.

- Fats: Choose healthy fats found in avocados, nuts, seeds, and olive oil. These fats support brain function, absorb certain vitamins, and contribute to satiety.

Portion Control and Meal Composition:

Balancing these macronutrients while keeping within a 1200-calorie limit involves thoughtful portioning:

- **Protein Portion:** Aim for a palm-sized portion of protein in each meal.

- **Carbohydrates:** Fill a quarter of your plate with complex carbs, such as veggies or whole grains.

- **Healthy Fats:** Incorporate a small serving of healthy fats to add flavor and satiety to your meals.

Sample Meal Ideas:

Let's get creative with these balanced meal ideas:

-**Breakfast:** Greek yogurt with berries and a sprinkle of almonds or a veggie omelet with whole-grain toast.

- **Lunch:** Grilled chicken salad with mixed greens, quinoa, and a drizzle of olive oil-based dressing.

- **Dinner:** Baked salmon with roasted vegetables and a side of brown rice.

- **Snacks:** Hummus with carrot sticks, apple slices with almond butter, or a handful of nuts and seeds.

Hydration and Mindful Eating:

Remember, it's important to stay hydrated. Fortify your body with water, herbal teas, or infused water to avoid mindless munching.

Finally, learn to eat mindfully. To truly enjoy your meals, pay attention to your body's hunger cues, taste every bite, and eat deliberately.

PORTION CONTROL TIPS

Portion control is knowing the right serving sizes to make sure you obtain the nutrients your body needs while controlling your calorie intake, rather than just restricting the amount of food you eat. By using this technique, you can savor a range of cuisines without going overboard.

Important Advice on Portion Control:

1. **Use Measuring Tools:** Make an investment in a kitchen scale, measuring cups, and spoons. When starting out on your journey, these tools are very helpful for precisely measuring portion sizes.

2. **Visual References:** Familiarize yourself with visual cues for portion sizes. For instance, a serving of meat is

about the size of a deck of cards, a cup of pasta or rice is roughly the size of a tennis ball, and a teaspoon of oil matches the tip of your thumb.

3. Plate Composition: Visualize your plate divided into sections: half for non-starchy vegetables, a quarter for lean proteins, and the remaining quarter for whole grains or starchy foods. This method helps maintain a balanced intake.

4. Mindful Eating: Slow down and savor each bite. Pay attention to hunger cues and stop eating when you feel comfortably full, not overstuffed.

5. Pre-portion Snacks: Avoid mindlessly snacking from large packages. Instead, pre-portion snacks into smaller bags or containers to prevent overeating.

6. Read Labels: Get acquainted with food labels to understand serving sizes and calorie content. This knowledge empowers better decision-making while grocery shopping.

7. Practice Moderation: You don't have to eliminate favorite foods entirely. Instead, enjoy them in moderation and adjust portion sizes accordingly.

Adopting Portion Control for Success:

A 1200-calorie diet's key to reaching your weight loss and health objectives is adopting portion management. It creates a more positive relationship with food, permits flexibility, and encourages mindful eating.

Recall that progress, not perfection, is the goal of this trip. As you make decisions, use these portion control suggestions as a guide, and acknowledge each accomplishment on the path to a better, happier you.

CHAPTER 3 : HIGH-PROTEIN RECIPES

BREAKFAST IDEAS

<u>1. Spinach and Feta Egg Muffins</u>

Prep/Cook Time:

25 minutes

Nutritional Info: (Per serving - 2 muffins)

- Calories: 170

- Protein: 14g

- Carbohydrates: 2g

- Fat: 11g

Ingredients:

- 6 large eggs

- 1 cup chopped spinach

- 1/4 cup crumbled feta cheese

- Salt and pepper to taste

Instructions:

1. Preheat the oven to 350°F (175°C) and grease a muffin tin.

2. In a bowl, whisk together the eggs, spinach, feta, salt, and pepper.

3. Pour the mixture evenly into the muffin cups.

4. Bake for 15-20 minutes or until the muffins are set.

5. Allow them to cool slightly before removing from the tin.

2. Greek Yogurt Parfait

Prep/Cook Time:

5 minutes

Nutritional Info:

- Calories: 240

- Protein: 18g

- Carbohydrates: 20g

- Fat: 10g

Ingredients:

- 1 cup Greek yogurt

- 1/2 cup mixed berries

- 2 tablespoons chopped nuts (almonds, walnuts, or pecans)

- 1 tablespoon honey (optional)

Instructions:

1. In a glass or bowl, layer Greek yogurt, mixed berries, and chopped nuts.

2. Drizzle honey on top if desired.

3. Turkey and Veggie Breakfast Skillet

Prep/Cook Time:

15 minutes

Nutritional Info:

- Calories: 220

- Protein: 22g

- Carbohydrates: 6g

- Fat: 12g

Ingredients:

- 4 oz. lean ground turkey

- 1/2 cup diced bell peppers

- 1/4 cup diced onion

- 1 teaspoon olive oil

- Salt, pepper, and preferred seasonings

Instructions:

1. Heat olive oil in a skillet over medium heat.

2. Add diced onion and bell peppers, sauté until softened.

3. Add ground turkey, breaking it up with a spatula, and cook until browned.

4. Season with salt, pepper, or preferred spices.

4. Quinoa Breakfast Bowl

Prep/Cook Time:

10 minutes

Nutritional Info:

- Calories: 290

- Protein: 15g

- Carbohydrates: 30g

- Fat: 13g

Ingredients:

- 1/2 cup cooked quinoa

- 1/4 cup cottage cheese

- 1 tablespoon chia seeds

- 1/2 cup sliced strawberries

- 1 tablespoon almond butter

Instructions:

1. In a bowl, layer cooked quinoa, cottage cheese, and chia seeds.

2. Top with sliced strawberries and a dollop of almond butter.

5. High-Protein Oatmeal

Prep/Cook Time:

10 minutes

Nutritional Info:

- Calories: 340

- Protein: 25g

- Carbohydrates: 40g

- Fat: 10g

Ingredients:

- 1/2 cup rolled oats

- 1 cup unsweetened almond milk

- 1 scoop protein powder (vanilla or chocolate)

- 1 tablespoon chia seeds

- 1/2 banana, sliced

- Optional: cinnamon, nuts, or berries for topping

Instructions:

1. In a saucepan, combine oats and almond milk. Cook over medium heat until oats are tender.

2. Stir in protein powder and chia seeds until well combined.

3. Transfer to a bowl, top with banana slices and preferred toppings.

LUNCH CREATIONS

1. Grilled Chicken Salad with Quinoa

Prep & Cooking Time:

- Prep: 10 minutes

- Cooking: 10-12 minutes

Nutritional Information (per serving):

- Calories: 320

- Protein: 30g

- Carbohydrates: 17g

- Fat: 14g

- Fiber: 4g

Ingredients:

- 4 oz boneless, skinless chicken breast

- 1/4 cup cooked quinoa

- 2 cups mixed greens

- 1/4 cup cherry tomatoes, halved

- 1/4 cucumber, sliced

- 1 tablespoon olive oil

- 1 tablespoon balsamic vinegar

- Salt and pepper to taste

Instructions:

1. Season the chicken breast with salt and pepper. Grill or pan-sear until fully cooked, about 5-6 minutes per side. Let it rest before slicing.

2. In a bowl, mix the cooked quinoa, mixed greens, cherry tomatoes, and cucumber.

3. Whisk together olive oil and balsamic vinegar for the dressing.

4. Top the salad with sliced chicken and drizzle with the prepared dressing.

Tuna and White Bean Salad

Prep & Cooking Time:

- Prep: 10 minutes

Nutritional Information (per serving):

- Calories: 280

- Protein: 28g

- Carbohydrates: 22g

- Fat: 10g

- Fiber: 7g

Ingredients:

- 1 can (5 oz) tuna, drained

- 1 cup cooked white beans

- 1/4 red onion, finely chopped

- 1 celery stalk, diced

- 1 tablespoon chopped parsley

- 1 tablespoon lemon juice

- 1 tablespoon olive oil

- Salt and pepper to taste

Instructions:

1. In a bowl, combine tuna, white beans, red onion, celery, and parsley.

2. Mix in lemon juice and olive oil. Season with salt and pepper.

3. Serve chilled.

Turkey and Avocado Wrap

Prep & Cooking Time:

- Prep: 5 minutes

Nutritional Information (per serving):

- Calories: 340

- Protein: 30g

- Carbohydrates: 28g

- Fat: 14g

- Fiber: 8g

Ingredients:

- 4 oz sliced turkey breast

- 1 whole grain wrap

- 1/4 avocado, mashed

- 1/2 cup spinach leaves

- 1/4 cup shredded carrots

- 1 tablespoon Greek yogurt

- 1 teaspoon Dijon mustard

Instructions:

1. Spread mashed avocado on the wrap. Layer with turkey slices, spinach, and shredded carrots.

2. Mix Greek yogurt and Dijon mustard, drizzle over the filling.

3. Roll up tightly and slice in half.

Salmon and Quinoa Stuffed Bell Peppers

Prep & Cooking Time:

- Prep: 15 minutes

- Cooking: 20-25 minutes

Nutritional Information (per serving):

- Calories: 320

- Protein: 28g

- Carbohydrates: 20g

- Fat: 14g

- Fiber: 4g

Ingredients:

- 2 bell peppers, halved and deseeded

- 6 oz cooked salmon, flaked

- 1/2 cup cooked quinoa

- 1/4 cup diced tomatoes

- 1/4 cup chopped spinach

- 1 tablespoon grated Parmesan cheese

- 1 teaspoon olive oil

- Salt and pepper to taste

Instructions:

1. Preheat oven to 375°F (190°C).

2. In a bowl, mix salmon, quinoa, diced tomatoes, chopped spinach, Parmesan, olive oil, salt, and pepper.

3. Stuff the bell pepper halves with the mixture.

4. Place on a baking sheet and bake for 20-25 minutes until peppers are tender.

Egg Salad Lettuce Wraps

Prep & Cooking Time:

- Prep: 10 minutes

Nutritional Information (per serving):

- Calories: 250

- Protein: 20g

- Carbohydrates: 5g

- Fat: 16g

- Fiber: 2g

Ingredients:

- 4 hard-boiled eggs, chopped

- 2 tablespoons plain Greek yogurt

- 1 tablespoon chopped chives

- 1 tablespoon Dijon mustard

- Lettuce leaves for wrapping

Instructions:

1. In a bowl, combine chopped eggs, Greek yogurt, chives, and Dijon mustard. Mix well.

2. Spoon the egg salad onto lettuce leaves.

3. Roll up the lettuce to create wraps.

DINNER DELIGHTS

1. Grilled Chicken and Quinoa Bowl

Prep & Cooking Time:

30 minutes

Nutritional Info: (Approx. per serving)

Calories: 450

Protein: 40g

Carbs: 35g

Fat: 15g

Ingredients:

- 6 oz boneless, skinless chicken breast

- 1/2 cup quinoa, uncooked

- 1 cup broccoli florets

- 1 tablespoon olive oil

- 1 teaspoon garlic powder

- Salt and pepper to taste

Instructions:

1. Marinate chicken with olive oil, garlic powder, salt, and pepper.

2. Grill chicken until fully cooked.

3. Cook quinoa according to package instructions.

4. Steam broccoli until tender-crisp.

5. Assemble the bowl with quinoa, sliced grilled chicken, and broccoli.

2. Baked Salmon with Asparagus

Prep & Cooking Time:

25 minutes

Nutritional Info: (Approx. per serving)

Calories: 380

Protein: 35g

Carbs: 10g

Fat: 20g

Ingredients:

- 8 oz salmon fillet

- 1 bunch asparagus spears

- 1 tablespoon lemon juice

- 1 teaspoon dill

- Salt and pepper to taste

Instructions:

1. Preheat oven to 400°F (200°C).

2. Place salmon on a baking sheet, drizzle with lemon juice, and sprinkle with dill, salt, and pepper.

3. Arrange asparagus around the salmon.

4. Bake for 15-20 minutes or until salmon is cooked through.

3. Turkey and Vegetable Stir-Fry

Prep & Cooking Time:

25 minutes

Nutritional Info: (Approx. per serving)

Calories: 420

Protein: 30g

Carbs: 15g

Fat: 25g

Ingredients:

- 1 lb ground turkey
- 2 cups mixed stir-fry vegetables (bell peppers, snap peas, carrots)
- 2 tablespoons soy sauce
- 1 tablespoon sesame oil
- 1 teaspoon ginger, minced
- 2 cloves garlic, minced

Instructions:

1. In a pan, cook ground turkey until browned.
2. Add minced ginger and garlic, stir until fragrant.
3. Add vegetables and cook until tender.
4. Stir in soy sauce and sesame oil.
5. Serve over cauliflower rice or steamed broccoli.

4. Lentil and Chickpea Salad

Prep & Cooking Time:

15 minutes

Nutritional Info: (Approx. per serving)

Calories: 380

Protein: 20g

Carbs: 45g

Fat: 15g

Ingredients:

- 1 cup cooked lentils

- 1 cup cooked chickpeas

- 1 cucumber, diced

- 1 cup cherry tomatoes, halved

- 1/4 cup feta cheese, crumbled

- 2 tablespoons olive oil

- 1 tablespoon balsamic vinegar

- Salt and pepper to taste

Instructions:

1. In a large bowl, combine lentils, chickpeas, cucumber, and cherry tomatoes.

2. Whisk together olive oil, balsamic vinegar, salt, and pepper.

3. Toss the salad with the dressing and sprinkle feta on top.

5. Shrimp and Zucchini Noodles

Prep & Cooking Time:

20 minutes

Nutritional Info: (Approx. per serving)

Calories: 300

Protein: 25g

Carbs: 15g

Fat: 15g

Ingredients:

- 8 oz shrimp, peeled and deveined

- 2 medium zucchinis, spiralized

- 2 tablespoons pesto sauce

- 1 tablespoon lemon juice

- 1 teaspoon red pepper flakes (optional)

- Salt and pepper to taste

Instructions:

1. Sauté shrimp in a pan until cooked.

2. Add zucchini noodles, pesto sauce, lemon juice, and red pepper flakes.

3. Cook until zucchini noodles are tender.

4. Season with salt and pepper.

SNACKS AND SMOOTHIES

Protein-Packed Greek Yogurt Parfait

Prep/Cook Time:

5 minutes

Nutritional Info (per serving):

- Calories: 250

- Protein: 20g

- Carbohydrates: 30g

- Fiber: 6g

- Fat: 8g

Ingredients:

- 1 cup non-fat Greek yogurt

- 1/2 cup fresh mixed berries (strawberries, blueberries, raspberries)

- 1 tablespoon honey or agave nectar

- 2 tablespoons chopped nuts (almonds, walnuts)

- 1 tablespoon chia seeds

Instructions:

1. In a bowl or glass, layer Greek yogurt, mixed berries, and a drizzle of honey/agave.

2. Sprinkle chopped nuts and chia seeds on top.

3. Repeat layering for a visually appealing parfait.

4. Serve immediately or refrigerate for later.

Green Protein Smoothie

Prep/Cook Time:

 5 minutes

Nutritional Info (per serving):

- Calories: 280

- Protein: 25g

- Carbohydrates: 20g

- Fiber: 5g

- Fat: 10g

Ingredients:

- 1 cup unsweetened almond milk

- 1 scoop vanilla protein powder

- 1/2 frozen banana

- 1 cup fresh spinach leaves

- 1 tablespoon almond butter

- Ice cubes (optional)

Instructions:

1. Blend almond milk, protein powder, frozen banana, spinach, and almond butter until smooth.

2. Add ice cubes if desired for a cooler consistency.

3. Pour into a glass and serve immediately.

Tuna and Avocado Salad

Prep/Cook Time:

10 minutes

Nutritional Info (per serving):

- Calories: 280

- Protein: 30g

- Carbohydrates: 10g

- Fiber: 7g

- Fat: 15g

Ingredients:

- 1 can (5 oz) tuna, drained

- 1/2 ripe avocado, diced

- 1 tablespoon chopped red onion

- 1 tablespoon chopped cilantro

- Juice of 1/2 lime

- Salt and pepper to taste

Instructions:

1. In a bowl, combine tuna, diced avocado, red onion, cilantro, lime juice, salt, and pepper.

2. Mix gently until well combined.

3. Serve as a salad or on whole-grain crackers.

<u>**Berry Protein Smoothie Bowl**</u>

Prep/Cook Time:

5 minutes

Nutritional Info (per serving):

- Calories: 300

- Protein: 25g

- Carbohydrates: 35g

- Fiber: 8g

- Fat: 5g

Ingredients:

- 1 cup frozen mixed berries

- 1/2 cup non-fat Greek yogurt

- 1 scoop protein powder (vanilla or berry flavor)

- 2 tablespoons granola

- Fresh berries for topping

Instructions:

1. Blend frozen berries, Greek yogurt, and protein powder until smooth.

2. Pour into a bowl and top with granola and fresh berries.

<u>**Cottage Cheese and Veggie Dip**</u>

Prep/Cook Time:

10 minutes

Nutritional Info (per serving):

- Calories: 220

- Protein: 28g

- Carbohydrates: 12g

- Fiber: 2g

- Fat: 6g

Ingredients:

- 1 cup low-fat cottage cheese

- 1/4 cup diced cucumber

- 1/4 cup diced bell peppers (assorted colors)

- 1 tablespoon chopped fresh dill

- 1/2 teaspoon garlic powder

- Salt and pepper to taste

Instructions:

1. In a food processor, blend cottage cheese, cucumber, bell peppers, dill, garlic powder, salt, and pepper until smooth.

2. Serve as a dip with sliced vegetables or whole-grain crackers.

CHAPTER 4 : LOW CARB WONDERS

CARB SUSTITUTES AND ALTERNATIVES

1. Cauliflower Pizza Crust

Prep and Cooking Time:

40-45 minutes

Nutritional Info (per serving):

- Calories: 180

- Protein: 14g

- Fat: 9g

- Carbohydrates: 10g

- Fiber: 4g

Ingredients:

- 1 medium-sized cauliflower head

- 1 egg

- ½ cup grated Parmesan cheese

- 1 teaspoon dried oregano

- ½ teaspoon garlic powder

- Salt and pepper to taste

- Tomato sauce, cheese, and toppings of choice

Instructions:

1. Preheat oven to 400°F (200°C). Line a baking sheet with parchment paper.

2. Cut the cauliflower into florets and pulse in a food processor until it resembles rice.

3. Microwave the cauliflower rice for 5-6 minutes. Let it cool.

4. Place the cooled cauliflower rice in a clean kitchen towel and squeeze out excess moisture.

5. In a bowl, combine cauliflower, egg, Parmesan, oregano, garlic powder, salt, and pepper. Mix well.

6. Spread the mixture onto the prepared baking sheet, shaping it into a pizza crust.

7. Bake for 20-25 minutes or until golden and crisp.

8. Add your desired tomato sauce, cheese, and toppings. Return to the oven for 5-7 minutes or until the cheese melts.

2. Zucchini Noodles (Zoodles) with Pesto

Prep and Cooking Time:

10-12 minutes

Nutritional Info (per serving):

- Calories: 120

- Protein: 3g

- Fat: 10g

- Carbohydrates: 6g

- Fiber: 2g

Ingredients:

- 4 medium zucchinis

- 2 tablespoons olive oil

- ⅓ cup basil pesto

- Salt and pepper to taste

- Optional: grated Parmesan cheese

Instructions:

1. Spiralize the zucchinis into noodle shapes.

2. Heat olive oil in a pan over medium heat.

3. Add zucchini noodles and sauté for 2-3 minutes until tender.

4. Stir in the basil pesto and cook for an additional minute.

5. Season with salt and pepper. Top with grated Parmesan if desired.

3. Portobello Mushroom Bun Burgers

Prep and Cooking Time:

20-25 minutes

Nutritional Info (per serving):

- Calories: 250

- Protein: 30g

- Fat: 10g

- Carbohydrates: 5g

- Fiber: 2g

Ingredients:

- 4 large portobello mushrooms

- 1 pound ground turkey or beef

- Salt and pepper to taste

- Toppings of choice (lettuce, tomato, cheese)

Instructions:

1. Remove the stems from the portobello mushrooms and gently scrape out the gills.

2. Season the mushroom caps with salt and pepper.

3. Grill or pan-fry the mushrooms for 4-5 minutes on each side.

4. Form the ground turkey or beef into burger patties and cook according to preference.

5. Assemble the burgers using the portobello mushrooms as buns and add desired toppings.

4. Eggplant Lasagna

Prep and Cooking Time:

60-70 minutes

Nutritional Info (per serving):

- Calories: 320

- Protein: 24g

- Fat: 20g

- Carbohydrates: 10g

- Fiber: 4g

Ingredients:

- 1 large eggplant, sliced lengthwise

- 1 pound ground beef or turkey

- 1 cup marinara sauce

- 1 cup ricotta cheese

- 1 cup shredded mozzarella cheese

- 2 tablespoons olive oil

- Italian seasoning, salt, and pepper to taste

Instructions:

1. Preheat oven to 375°F (190°C).

2. Brush eggplant slices with olive oil, season with Italian seasoning, salt, and pepper. Roast for 15-20 minutes.

3. In a skillet, cook the ground beef or turkey until browned. Drain excess fat.

4. In a baking dish, layer marinara sauce, roasted eggplant slices, cooked meat, ricotta cheese, and mozzarella. Repeat layers.

5. Bake for 25-30 minutes until bubbly and cheese is golden brown.

5. Spaghetti Squash with Turkey Bolognese

Prep and Cooking Time:

60-65 minutes

Nutritional Info (per serving):

- Calories: 280

- Protein: 28g

- Fat: 12g

- Carbohydrates: 15g

- Fiber: 4g

Ingredients:

- 1 medium spaghetti squash

- 1 pound ground turkey

- 1 cup marinara sauce

- 2 cloves garlic, minced

- 2 tablespoons olive oil

- Salt, pepper, and Italian seasoning to taste

- Optional: grated Parmesan cheese

Instructions:

1. Preheat oven to 400°F (200°C).

2. Cut the spaghetti squash in half lengthwise and scoop out the seeds.

3. Brush the inside with olive oil and season with salt and pepper.

4. Place squash halves face-down on a baking sheet and roast for 40-45 minutes.

5. In a skillet, heat olive oil and sauté garlic until fragrant. Add ground turkey and cook until browned.

6. Stir in marinara sauce and simmer for 10-15 minutes.

7. Use a fork to scrape the cooked spaghetti squash into strands.

8. Serve the turkey bolognese over the spaghetti squash. Top with grated Parmesan if desired.

RECIPES WITH MINIMAL CARBS

Cabbage and Beef Stir-Fry

Prep & Cook Time:

20 minutes

Nutritional Info (per serving):

- Calories: 280

- Carbohydrates: 9g

- Protein: 25g

- Fat: 16g

Ingredients:

- 1 lb lean ground beef
- 1 small cabbage, thinly sliced
- 2 tablespoons soy sauce or tamari
- 2 cloves garlic, minced
- 1 teaspoon ginger, grated
- 2 green onions, chopped
- 1 tablespoon sesame oil
- Salt and pepper to taste

Instructions:

1. In a skillet, brown the ground beef over medium heat. Drain excess fat.

2. Add garlic, ginger, and sliced cabbage to the skillet. Stir-fry for 5-7 minutes until cabbage is tender.

3. Stir in soy sauce, sesame oil, green onions, salt, and pepper. Cook for an additional 2 minutes.

4. Serve hot.

Avocado and Tuna Salad

Prep Time:

10 minutes

Nutritional Info (per serving):

- Calories: 320

- Carbohydrates: 10g

- Protein: 20g

- Fat: 24g

Ingredients:

- 2 cans (5 oz each) tuna, drained

- 2 ripe avocados, diced

- ½ red onion, finely chopped

- 1 celery stalk, finely chopped

- Juice of 1 lime

- 2 tablespoons olive oil

- Salt and pepper to taste

- Fresh parsley (optional, for garnish)

Instructions:

1. In a bowl, mix tuna, diced avocado, red onion, and celery.

2. Drizzle with lime juice and olive oil. Season with salt and pepper.

3. Gently toss to combine.

4. Garnish with fresh parsley if desired and serve chilled.

Spaghetti Squash with Tomato Basil Sauce

Prep & Cook Time:

60 minutes

Nutritional Info (per serving):

- Calories: 220

- Carbohydrates: 32g

- Protein: 3g

- Fat: 10g

Ingredients:

- 1 medium spaghetti squash

- 2 cups tomato basil sauce (sugar-free)

- 1 tablespoon olive oil

- Fresh basil leaves for garnish

- Salt and pepper to taste

Instructions:

1. Preheat oven to 375°F (190°C).

2. Cut spaghetti squash in half lengthwise and scoop out the seeds.

3. Drizzle olive oil over the squash halves and sprinkle with salt and pepper.

4. Place squash halves on a baking sheet, cut side down, and bake for 40-45 minutes until tender.

5. Scrape the squash flesh with a fork to create "spaghetti."

6. Serve with warmed tomato basil sauce and garnish with fresh basil leaves.

<u>Chicken Broccoli Alfredo</u>

Prep & Cook Time:

30 minutes

Nutritional Info (per serving):

- Calories: 380

- Carbohydrates: 8g

- Protein: 28g

- Fat: 26g

Ingredients:

- 2 boneless, skinless chicken breasts

- 2 cups broccoli florets

- 1 cup heavy cream

- ½ cup grated Parmesan cheese

- 2 cloves garlic, minced

- 2 tablespoons butter

- Salt and pepper to taste

Instructions:

1. Season chicken breasts with salt and pepper. Grill or cook in a skillet until done. Slice into strips.

2. In a saucepan, melt butter and sauté garlic for 1 minute.

3. Add heavy cream and Parmesan cheese, stirring until the cheese melts and the sauce thickens.

4. Blanch broccoli in boiling water for 2 minutes, then drain.

5. Combine chicken, broccoli, and Alfredo sauce in a pan. Heat through and serve hot.

Greek Salad with Grilled Chicken

Prep & Cook Time:

25 minutes

Nutritional Info (per serving):

- Calories: 340

- Carbohydrates: 9g

- Protein: 30g

- Fat: 20g

Ingredients:

- 2 boneless, skinless chicken breasts

- 4 cups mixed greens

- ½ cucumber, sliced

- ½ red onion, thinly sliced

- 1 cup cherry tomatoes, halved

- ½ cup crumbled feta cheese

- ¼ cup Kalamata olives

- 2 tablespoons olive oil

- 2 tablespoons red wine vinegar

- 1 teaspoon dried oregano

- Salt and pepper to taste

Instructions:

1. Season chicken breasts with salt, pepper, and oregano. Grill until fully cooked.

2. In a large bowl, combine mixed greens, cucumber, red onion, cherry tomatoes, feta cheese, and olives.

3. In a small bowl, whisk together olive oil and red wine vinegar to make the dressing.

4. Slice grilled chicken and add it to the salad. Drizzle with the dressing and toss gently to coat.

MAINTAINING ENERGY LEVELS WITHOUT CARBS

Cutting back on carbohydrates is a common first step in weight loss, but it doesn't have to mean sacrificing energy. Although carbohydrates are the main source of energy, there are many other nutrient-dense options that can help maintain vigor.

1. Embrace Healthy Fats: Incorporating healthy fats like avocados, nuts, seeds, and olive oil provides a steady source of energy. These fats are dense in calories but offer prolonged satiety and sustained energy without the spikes and crashes associated with high-carb meals.

2. Lean Proteins: Protein-rich foods such as lean meats, fish, eggs, and plant-based sources like tofu and legumes not only aid in muscle repair but also offer a steady energy supply. Protein takes longer to digest, keeping you fuller for longer and providing a stable energy release.

3. Fiber-Rich Foods: Opt for fibrous vegetables, berries, and whole grains. While some contain carbohydrates, their high fiber content slows down digestion, preventing rapid spikes in blood sugar levels and providing sustained energy.

4. Strategic Meal Timing: Eating smaller, balanced meals throughout the day helps maintain consistent energy levels. Combining protein, healthy fats, and fiber in each meal can prevent energy crashes and keep you feeling alert and focused.

5. Stay Hydrated: Dehydration can lead to fatigue. Ensure adequate water intake throughout the day to support metabolic processes and maintain energy levels.

6. Mindful Snacking: When snacking, choose wisely. Nuts, Greek yogurt, cheese, and vegetable sticks with hummus can provide a boost without the need for refined carbohydrates.

7. Prioritize Sleep and Exercise: Quality sleep and regular physical activity play crucial roles in sustaining energy levels. Aim for adequate rest and engage in moderate exercise to enhance endurance and vitality.

Through a varied diet and an emphasis on foods that provide long-lasting energy, you can continue to feel energetic all day long even as you cut back on your consumption of carbohydrates. Recall that the secret to maximizing energy levels during a weight loss journey is balance and variety.

CHAPTER 5 : HIGHER FIBER DELICACIES

IMPORTANCE OF FIBER IN WEIGHT LOSS

Fiber is a secret weapon in your weight loss quest, not merely for maintaining the health of your digestive system. The importance of fiber in the fight to lose weight and feel your best cannot be emphasized.

The following explains why fiber is your reliable ally in the fight against excess weight:

1. **Control of Appetite and Satiety:** Fiber-rich foods take longer to digest, which prolongs the sense of fullness and satisfaction. Fiber-rich meals and snacks naturally help reduce overall calorie consumption, which is a key component of weight management, by squelching hunger cravings.

2. **Blood Sugar Stabilization:** By reducing the rate at which sugar is absorbed, fiber helps control blood sugar levels and avoids sudden spikes and dips in energy. Better control over cravings and impulsive eating is facilitated by this steady flow of energy.

3. Boosting Metabolism: Certain types of fiber, like soluble fiber found in oats, beans, and fruits, have been linked to a slight increase in metabolism. While the effect might be modest, every bit counts on your weight loss journey.

4. Digestive Health: A healthy gut is crucial for overall well-being. Fiber promotes a healthy digestive system, preventing constipation and ensuring proper bowel movements, which can indirectly support weight loss by maintaining optimal digestive function.

5. Reducing Calorie Absorption: In the digestive tract, fiber binds to some calories and fats, which lessens the body's absorption of these substances. Although it's not a magic cure, this can help make the weight loss process go more smoothly.

It is actually quite easy to include fiber in your meals. Give special attention to complete, unprocessed foods such as whole grains, legumes, nuts, seeds, fruits, and vegetables. These nutrient-dense foods include a variety of vitamins, minerals, and antioxidants that are vital for good health in addition to fiber.

Never undervalue the importance of fiber in your quest for a healthier, more trimmer self. It's essential to effective and long-lasting weight loss, not just a way to control digestion. Accept meals high in fiber and see how they can revolutionize both your overall health and your attempts to lose weight.

FIBER RICH MEAL OPTIONS

Quinoa and Black Bean Salad

Prep/Cook Time:

20 minutes

Nutritional Info (per serving):

- Calories: 320

- Protein: 12g

- Carbohydrates: 50g

- Fiber: 12g

- Fat: 8g

Ingredients:

- 1 cup cooked quinoa

- 1 can (15 oz) black beans (drained and rinsed)

- 1 cup diced tomatoes

- 1/2 cup diced red bell pepper

- 1/4 cup chopped cilantro

- 2 tablespoons lime juice

- 1 tablespoon olive oil

- Salt and pepper to taste

Instructions:

1. In a bowl, mix quinoa, black beans, tomatoes, bell pepper, and cilantro.

2. In a separate small bowl, whisk lime juice, olive oil, salt, and pepper.

3. Pour the dressing over the salad and toss gently to combine.

4. Serve chilled.

Chickpea and Vegetable Stir-Fry

Prep/Cook Time:

15 minutes

Nutritional Info (per serving):

- Calories: 280

- Protein: 10g

- Carbohydrates: 38g

- Fiber: 10g

- Fat: 9g

Ingredients:

- 1 can (15 oz) chickpeas (drained and rinsed)

- 2 cups mixed vegetables (broccoli, bell peppers, snap peas)
- 2 cloves garlic (minced)
- 2 tablespoons low-sodium soy sauce
- 1 tablespoon sesame oil
- 1 teaspoon ginger (minced)
- Cooked brown rice (optional)

Instructions:

1. Heat sesame oil in a pan, add garlic and ginger, sauté for a minute.

2. Add mixed vegetables and chickpeas, stir-fry until vegetables are tender.

3. Pour soy sauce over the mixture, stir well, and cook for another 2 minutes.

4. Serve alone or over brown rice.

Certainly, here are more fiber-rich meal options for your 1200-calorie diet cookbook:

Spinach and Lentil Soup

Prep/Cook Time:

30 minutes

Nutritional Info (per serving):

- Calories: 260
- Protein: 18g

- Carbohydrates: 40g

- Fiber: 15g

- Fat: 1g

Ingredients:

- 1 cup dried lentils (rinsed)

- 4 cups vegetable broth

- 2 cups chopped spinach

- 1 onion (diced)

- 2 cloves garlic (minced)

- 1 teaspoon cumin

- Salt and pepper to taste

Instructions:

1. In a pot, sauté onion and garlic until softened.

2. Add lentils, vegetable broth, and cumin. Bring to a boil, then simmer for 20 minutes.

3. Stir in chopped spinach and cook for an additional 5 minutes.

4. Season with salt and pepper.

Grilled Vegetable and Quinoa Bowl

Prep/Cook Time:

25 minutes

Nutritional Info (per serving):

- Calories: 280

- Protein: 10g

- Carbohydrates: 40g

- Fiber: 8g

- Fat: 8g

Ingredients:

- 1 cup cooked quinoa

- 2 cups mixed grilled vegetables (zucchini, bell peppers, eggplant)

- 2 tablespoons balsamic vinaigrette

- 1/4 cup crumbled feta cheese (optional)

- Fresh basil leaves (for garnish)

Instructions:

1. Toss grilled vegetables with balsamic vinaigrette.

2. Place quinoa in a bowl, top with grilled vegetables.

3. Sprinkle with feta cheese and garnish with basil leaves.

Avocado and Black Bean Wrap

Prep/Cook Time:

10 minutes

Nutritional Info (per serving):

- Calories: 290

- Protein: 10g

- Carbohydrates: 38g

- Fiber: 12g

- Fat: 12g

Ingredients:

- 1 whole wheat tortilla

- 1/2 avocado (sliced)

- 1/2 cup black beans (cooked or canned)

- 1/4 cup diced tomatoes

- 2 tablespoons chopped red onion

- 1 tablespoon lime juice

- Handful of baby spinach

Instructions:

1. In a bowl, mix black beans, diced tomatoes, red onion, and lime juice.

2. Spread avocado on the tortilla, add the bean mixture and baby spinach.

3. Roll the tortilla into a wrap.

Mediterranean Quinoa Salad

Prep/Cook Time:

15 minutes

Nutritional Info (per serving):

- Calories: 310

- Protein: 8g

- Carbohydrates: 38g

- Fiber: 6g

- Fat: 14g

Ingredients:

- 1 cup cooked quinoa

- 1 cucumber (diced)

- 1 cup cherry tomatoes (halved)

- 1/4 cup chopped red onion

- 1/4 cup chopped fresh parsley

- 2 tablespoons olive oil

- 2 tablespoons lemon juice

- Feta cheese crumbles (optional)

Instructions:

1. In a large bowl, combine quinoa, cucumber, cherry tomatoes, red onion, and parsley.

2. Drizzle olive oil and lemon juice over the mixture, toss to combine.

3. Sprinkle with feta cheese if desired.

SNACK IDEAS PACKED WITH FIBER

Avocado and Black Bean Dip

Preparation Time:

10 minutes

Nutritional Info: (per serving)

  - Calories: 120

  - Fiber: 7g

  - Protein: 5g

Ingredients:

  - 1 ripe avocado

  - 1 can (15 oz) black beans, drained and rinsed

  - 1 lime (juiced)

  - 1 clove garlic, minced

  - Salt and pepper to taste

Instructions:

  1. In a food processor, combine avocado, black beans, lime juice, garlic, salt, and pepper.

  2. Blend until smooth.

  3. Serve with sliced veggies or whole-grain crackers.

Greek Yogurt Parfait

Preparation Time:

5 minutes

Nutritional Info: (per serving)

  - Calories: 250

  - Fiber: 5g

- Protein: 18g

Ingredients:

- 1 cup Greek yogurt
- 1/2 cup mixed berries
- 2 tablespoons granola
- 1 tablespoon honey (optional)

Instructions:

1. Layer Greek yogurt, mixed berries, granola, and honey (if desired) in a glass.
2. Repeat layers.
3. Serve chilled.

Chickpea Salad

Preparation Time:

15 minutes

Nutritional Info: (per serving)

- Calories: 220
- Fiber: 8g
- Protein: 7g

Ingredients:

- 1 can (15 oz) chickpeas, drained and rinsed
- 1 cucumber, diced

- 1 bell pepper, diced

- 1/4 cup red onion, finely chopped

- 2 tablespoons olive oil

- 2 tablespoons lemon juice

- Fresh parsley (chopped)

- Salt and pepper to taste

Instructions:

1. In a bowl, combine chickpeas, cucumber, bell pepper, and red onion.

2. Drizzle olive oil and lemon juice over the mixture.

3. Season with salt, pepper, and chopped parsley. Toss gently.

4. Serve chilled.

Apple Slices with Almond Butter

Preparation Time:

3 minutes

Nutritional Info: (per serving)

- Calories: 180

- Fiber: 6g

- Protein: 4g

Ingredients:

- 1 apple, sliced

- 2 tablespoons almond butter

Instructions:

1. Spread almond butter on apple slices.

2. Enjoy as a tasty and quick snack.

<u>Quinoa and Veggie Stuffed Bell Peppers</u>

Preparation Time:

35 minutes

Nutritional Info: (per serving)

- Calories: 220

- Fiber: 8g

- Protein: 9g

Ingredients:

- 2 bell peppers, halved and seeds removed

- 1 cup cooked quinoa

- 1/2 cup black beans (cooked or canned)

- 1/2 cup corn kernels (cooked or canned)

- 1/4 cup diced tomatoes

- 1/4 cup chopped cilantro

- 1 teaspoon cumin

- Salt and pepper to taste

Instructions:

1. Preheat oven to 375°F (190°C).

2. In a bowl, mix quinoa, black beans, corn, tomatoes, cilantro, cumin, salt, and pepper.

3. Stuff the halved bell peppers with the quinoa mixture.

4. Bake for 25-30 minutes until peppers are tender.

Hummus and Veggie Wraps

Preparation Time:

10 minutes

Nutritional Info: (per serving)

- Calories: 180

- Fiber: 6g

- Protein: 5g

Ingredients:

- Whole-grain tortillas

- 1/2 cup hummus

- Sliced cucumbers, bell peppers, and tomatoes

Instructions:

1. Spread hummus evenly on tortillas.

2. Add sliced veggies.

3. Roll up and slice into pinwheels.

Kale Chips

Preparation Time:

20 minutes

Nutritional Info: (per serving)

- Calories: 50

- Fiber: 2g

- Protein: 2g

Ingredients:

- 1 bunch kale, washed and dried

- 1 tablespoon olive oil

- Salt and pepper to taste

Instructions:

1. Preheat oven to 300°F (150°C).

2. Remove kale leaves from stems and tear into bite-sized pieces.

3. Massage olive oil into kale leaves and sprinkle with salt and pepper.

4. Spread kale on a baking sheet and bake for 10-15 minutes until crispy.

Edamame and Sea Salt

Preparation Time:

5 minutes

Nutritional Info: (per serving)

- Calories: 120

- Fiber: 9g

- Protein: 11g

Ingredients:

- 1 cup edamame (frozen or fresh)

- Sea salt to taste

Instructions:

1. Boil or steam edamame according to package instructions.

2. Sprinkle with sea salt and enjoy as a satisfying snack.

Berry and Chia Seed Pudding

Preparation Time:

15 minutes (+chilling time)

Nutritional Info: (per serving)

- Calories: 150

- Fiber: 10g

- Protein: 4g

Ingredients:

- 1/2 cup mixed berries (fresh or frozen)

- 2 tablespoons chia seeds

- 1 cup unsweetened almond milk

- 1 tablespoon honey (optional)

Instructions:

1. Mix chia seeds and almond milk in a jar or bowl. Stir well.

2. Let it sit for 10 minutes, stirring occasionally.

3. Layer chia pudding with mixed berries.

4. Drizzle with honey if desired.

Cottage Cheese and Pineapple Bowl

Preparation Time:

3 minutes

Nutritional Info: (per serving)

- Calories: 150

- Fiber: 2g

- Protein: 13g

Ingredients:

- 1/2 cup cottage cheese

- 1/2 cup pineapple chunks (fresh or canned)

Instructions:

1. Combine cottage cheese and pineapple chunks in a bowl.

2. Mix well and enjoy this refreshing and protein-packed snack.

CHAPTER 6 : MEAL PLANNING AND SAMPLE MENUS

WEEKLY MEAL PLANS

Meal planning is your secret weapon on the journey toward your weight loss goals. It's not just about what you eat; it's about intentional choices that set you up for success. With a well-thought-out plan, you'll navigate your week with ease, making healthier choices and staying on track.

Why Meal Planning Matters:

1. Consistency: Planning your meals allows you to maintain consistency in your dietary choices, ensuring you stick to your calorie and nutritional goals.

2. Saves Time and Effort: It eliminates the stress of figuring out what to eat each day. You'll save time on grocery shopping and food preparation.

3. Balanced Nutrition: By planning your meals in advance, you can ensure a balanced intake of nutrients, essential for sustaining your energy levels and overall health.

4. Reduces Temptations: With meals already planned, you're less likely to succumb to unhealthy, impulse food choices.

<u>Sample Weekly Meal Plan:</u>

Day 1:

- Breakfast: Greek Yogurt Parfait with Mixed Berries and Granola
- Lunch: Quinoa and Veggie Stuffed Bell Peppers
- Dinner: Baked Salmon with Steamed Broccoli and Cauliflower
- Snack: Apple Slices with Almond Butter

Day 2:

- Breakfast: Avocado and Black Bean Dip with Sliced Veggies
- Lunch: Chickpea Salad
- Dinner: Grilled Chicken Breast with Mixed Greens Salad
- Snack: Cottage Cheese and Pineapple Bowl

Day 3:

- Breakfast: Chia Seed Pudding with Berries
- Lunch: Hummus and Veggie Wraps
- Dinner: Turkey Meatballs with Zucchini Noodles

- Snack: Kale Chips

Day 4:

- Breakfast: Whole Grain Toast with Peanut Butter and Banana Slices

- Lunch: Lentil Soup with a Side Salad

- Dinner: Stir-Fried Tofu with Mixed Vegetables

- Snack: Edamame with Sea Salt

Day 5:

- Breakfast: Spinach and Feta Omelet

- Lunch: Tuna Salad Lettuce Wraps

- Dinner: Baked Cod with Roasted Asparagus

- Snack: Berry Smoothie (Greek Yogurt + Berries)

Day 6:

- Breakfast: Oatmeal with Berries and Almonds

- Lunch: Quinoa Salad with Avocado Dressing

- Dinner: Grilled Shrimp Skewers with Quinoa

- Snack: Carrot Sticks with Hummus

Day 7:

- Breakfast: Protein Pancakes with Fresh Fruit

- Lunch: Caprese Salad with Grilled Chicken Strips

- Dinner: Beef Stir-Fry with Brown Rice

- Snack: Greek Yogurt with Honey and Almonds

CHAPTER 7 : EXCERCISE AND LIFESTYLE SUPPORT

INCORPORATING EXCERCISE ROUTINES

Exercise is essential to taking care of your body and mind; it's not only about burning calories. It increases general fitness, strengthens muscles, and speeds up metabolism. Although our cookbook provides dietary guidance, combining it with a comprehensive fitness program enhances the outcomes.

Think about including a range of workouts that suit your tastes and way of living. Discover what motivates you to move, whether it's weight training, yoga, jogging, cycling, dancing, or brisk strolling. Build up your routine gradually, pay attention to your body, and start out slowly.

Setting Realistic Goals

Establishing attainable fitness objectives is essential. Consistency is more important than intensity. Start out small and work your way up to longer and more intense workouts. Recall that every step matters, whether you're working out at the gym, taking a quick stroll, or doing yoga.

Creating a Supportive Lifestyle

A comprehensive strategy for weight loss goes beyond diet and exercise. Your journey is greatly impacted by the lifestyle decisions you make. Pay attention to stress reduction, mindfulness, and restful sleep. While stress management encourages better choices and lowers emotional eating, getting enough sleep promotes healing and hormone regulation.

Building a Support System

Surround yourself with a supportive network. Share your goals with friends, family, or join communities focused on health and fitness. Having a supportive environment fosters motivation, encouragement, and accountability.

Adapting and Enjoying the Journey

Accept adaptability in your daily schedule. Because life can be unpredictable, it's acceptable to modify your plans. Recall that the goal of this journey is to nourish both your body and spirit. Enjoy the journey, acknowledge your tiny accomplishments, and treat yourself with kindness when you face obstacles.

MANAGING CRAVINGS AND SETBACKS

Understanding Cravings: Cravings often stem from various triggers—emotions, habits, or even physiological cues. Acknowledging and understanding these triggers is the first step in managing cravings. Don't perceive cravings as weaknesses; instead, see them as signals your body sends, telling you to pay attention.

Strategies for Managing Cravings:

- Mindful Eating: Practice mindful eating by savoring every bite. Engage your senses, appreciate flavors, and eat slowly. This allows your body to recognize fullness and satisfaction.

- Healthy Alternatives: Stock up on nutritious, satisfying alternatives to your usual cravings. Whether it's swapping chips for roasted nuts or indulging in dark chocolate instead of sugary treats, find healthier options that still hit the spot.

- Stay Hydrated: Sometimes, thirst can masquerade as hunger. Ensure you're adequately hydrated throughout the day to avoid unnecessary cravings.

- Plan Ahead: Plan your meals and snacks in advance. Having a structured eating plan helps in curbing impulsive eating and sticking to healthier choices.

Dealing with Setbacks: Setbacks are an inevitable part of any journey. They are not indicators of failure but opportunities for growth and learning. Here's how to navigate setbacks:

- Be Kind to Yourself: Practice self-compassion. Don't be too hard on yourself if you slip up. Instead, use setbacks as lessons to understand your triggers and develop better coping strategies.

- Revisit Your Goals: Remind yourself of why you started this journey. Revisit your goals and reaffirm your commitment. Adjust your approach if necessary but stay focused on the bigger picture.

- Seek Support: Reach out for support when faced with setbacks. Whether it's from friends, family, or a support group, having a network can provide encouragement and accountability.

CHAPTER 8 : TRACKING PROGRESS

MONITORING WEIGHT LOSS

Being able to see your success is one of the most empowering components of your weight loss journey. You can obtain useful insights into your accomplishments and places for growth by keeping track of and monitoring your efforts. Monitoring your progress involves more than just looking at numbers on a scale; it also involves appreciating each tiny victory and maintaining motivation as you work toward becoming a healthier version of yourself.

Why Track Progress?

- Motivation Boost: Tracking progress can serve as a source of motivation, providing tangible evidence of your hard work and dedication.

- Identifying Patterns: It helps in identifying patterns in your eating habits, exercise routine, and lifestyle that contribute positively or hinder your progress.

- Accountability: By holding yourself accountable, tracking allows you to stay committed to your goals.

Monitoring Weight Loss: Tips and Strategies

1. Use Multiple Metrics: While the scale is one tool, it's not the only measure of success. Consider measurements, body composition, clothing fit, energy levels, and overall well-being as additional markers of progress.

2. Consistency Matters: Establish a consistent tracking routine. Whether it's weekly weigh-ins, daily food journals, or regular measurements, consistency is key.

3. Set Realistic Goals: Break down your goals into smaller, achievable milestones. Celebrate each milestone reached to stay motivated.

4. Document and Reflect: Keep a journal or use an app to record your progress. Reflect on your successes and challenges, noting what works best for you.

5. Seek Support: Share your progress with a supportive friend, family member, or a community to stay accountable and encouraged.

Recall that your journey is distinct.

Everybody's experience with weight loss is different. There are times when progress isn't linear, and obstacles are a normal part of the journey. Accept the highs and lows and treat yourself with respect and resiliency. On your journey toward change, use your tracking data as a compass rather than as a yardstick.

You're actively contributing to your well-being when you make the commitment to track your progress. Your commitment and perseverance will open the door to long-lasting, beneficial adjustments that go far beyond scale measurements.

ADJUSTING THE PLAN

Here are some insightful tips on how to modify and enhance your weight loss program to guarantee ongoing success:

1. Monitoring Progress: Regularly assess your progress. Keep track of not just the number on the scale but also how you feel physically and emotionally. Notice the positive changes in energy levels, clothes fitting better, and improvements in overall well-being.

2. Listen to Your Body: Pay attention to your body's signals. If you're feeling fatigued, overly hungry, or experience any discomfort, it might be a sign that adjustments are necessary. Your body communicates its needs; tuning in and responding appropriately is key.

3. Plateau Breakers: Weight loss plateaus are common. If you hit a standstill, don't get discouraged. Consider adjusting your exercise routine, reassessing portion sizes, or introducing new foods to reignite progress.

4. Reassessing Caloric Needs: As your weight changes, your body's caloric needs may also shift. Consult with a healthcare professional or nutritionist to recalibrate your calorie intake accordingly.

5. Sustainable Changes: Aim for lasting lifestyle changes rather than quick fixes. Gradually incorporate new habits and maintain the ones that work best for you. Sustainable progress is about consistency and balance.

6. **Embrace Adaptability:** Your experience losing weight is distinct. Accept the freedom to modify the plan to fit your nutritional requirements, tastes, and way of life. Adjust meal times, make changes to recipes, and include new exercises that you find meaningful.

Keep in mind that making changes is a normal part of the process of becoming a healthier you. Accept these shifts as chances for development, education, and further advancement. Remain steadfast, exercise patience, and acknowledge each accomplishment, no matter how tiny.

You have all you need to succeed in your weight loss journey if you have perseverance, flexibility, and an optimistic outlook. The road to success isn't always straight.

CHAPTER 9 : FAQs AND TROUBLESHOOTING

COMMON QUESTIONS ANSWERED

1. Why Am I Not Losing Weight Despite Following the Diet?

- Troubleshooting: Ensure accurate portion control, check for hidden calories in condiments or beverages, reassess activity levels, and consult a healthcare professional for personalized advice.

2. Can I Substitute Ingredients in the Recipes?

- **Troubleshooting:** Yes, you can make substitutions, but be mindful of calorie and nutritional changes. Opt for healthier alternatives and adjust portion sizes accordingly.

3. I'm Always Hungry. What Should I Do?

- **Troubleshooting:** Increase fiber and protein intake, stay hydrated, eat smaller, more frequent meals, and include healthy fats for satiety.

4. Are Cheat Days Acceptable on This Diet?

- **Troubleshooting:** Occasional indulgences are fine but maintain moderation. Be mindful of portion sizes and don't let cheat days derail your overall progress.

5. How Can I Manage Cravings for Unhealthy Foods?

- **Troubleshooting:** Plan for healthier alternatives, practice mindful eating, keep unhealthy foods out of sight, and use portion-controlled servings if indulging occasionally.

6. I Feel Tired and Low on Energy. Any Suggestions?

- **Troubleshooting:** Ensure you're eating enough and staying hydrated. Include complex carbs for sustained energy, get enough sleep, and consider light exercise for a boost.

7. Can I Follow This Diet If I Have Dietary Restrictions (e.g., Vegetarian, Gluten-Free)?

- **Troubleshooting:** Yes, the diet can be adapted. There are plenty of options for various dietary preferences. Substitute ingredients to suit your needs.

8. How Can I Deal with Plateaus in Weight Loss?

- **Troubleshooting:** Reassess portion sizes, vary workouts, increase physical activity, and consider changing up your meal plan. Patience is crucial; plateaus are normal.

9. Is It Safe to Continue Exercising While Following a 1200-Calorie Diet?

- **Troubleshooting:** Exercise is generally safe but listen to your body. Adjust intensity and duration as needed. Consult a professional if feeling overly fatigued.

10. What Should I Do If I Feel Overwhelmed or Discouraged?

- **Troubleshooting:** Reach out to a support system, practice self-compassion, remind yourself of your goals and progress, and seek guidance or advice if needed.

11. Can I Drink Alcohol While Following This Diet?

- **Troubleshooting:** Alcohol contains empty calories and may hinder weight loss. Moderation is key; limit alcohol intake and be aware of its impact on your progress.

12. How Do I Stay Motivated Throughout the Diet?

- **Troubleshooting:** Set achievable goals, track progress, celebrate milestones, seek inspiration from success stories, and focus on the benefits beyond weight loss.

13. What Are Some Quick, Low-Calorie Snack Options?

- Troubleshooting: Opt for veggies with hummus, Greek yogurt with berries, rice cakes with nut butter, or a handful of nuts and seeds for quick, satisfying snacks.

14. How Do I Avoid Boredom with the Meal Plan?

- Troubleshooting: Experiment with new recipes, add variety with different spices and herbs, explore diverse cuisines, and involve family or friends in meal planning.

15. Is It Normal to Feel Frustrated with Slow Progress?

- Troubleshooting: Absolutely normal. Focus on the overall journey, not just the scale. Track non-scale victories like increased energy, better sleep, and improved mood.

OVERCOMING PLATEAUS

Plateaus are a common phase in weight loss, and they can occur for various reasons. Sometimes, it's your body's way of adjusting to the new calorie intake or exercise routine. Other times, it could be due to increased stress, lack of sleep, or hormonal fluctuations.

The good news? Plateaus are not permanent roadblocks; they are hurdles waiting to be conquered. Here are some strategies to help you break through and reignite your progress:

1. Reassess Your Approach: Take a step back and evaluate your eating habits, exercise routine, and overall lifestyle. Are there any changes you can make to stimulate your body's response? Tweaking your calorie intake, trying different workout routines, or incorporating new foods can sometimes kickstart progress.

2. Stay Mindful of Portions: It's easy to become complacent with portion sizes over time. Revisit your portion control strategies and ensure you're accurately measuring your food intake. Sometimes, recalibrating your portion sizes can make a significant difference.

3. Mix Up Your Workouts: Your body gets accustomed to repetitive exercises. Shake things up by trying new workouts, increasing intensity, or incorporating strength training to challenge different muscle groups.

4. Prioritize Rest and Recovery: Inadequate sleep and excessive stress can hinder weight loss progress. Focus on quality sleep and stress management techniques like meditation or yoga to support your body's overall well-being.

5. Patience and Persistence: Plateaus can test your patience, but remember, progress is not always linear. Celebrate non-scale victories like increased energy levels, improved stamina, or clothing fitting better to stay motivated.

CHAPTER 10 : CONCLUSION

FINAL WORDS OF ENCOURAGEMENT

Thank you for finishing "Lose 30lbs in 30 Days: Your 1200-Calorie Guide to Fast Weight Loss," which was an incredibly enlightening experience. Remember this as you turn the last page of this book: this is the start of a new, healthier, and more powerful chapter in your life.

To lose weight and embrace wellness, you've explored a world of nutrient-dense dishes, discovered mindful eating, and embraced the power of choice. You've found something deep, though, something that goes beyond the numbers on the scale: the inner strength to transform your life for the better.

Your dedication to a better, happier version of yourself is evident in your commitment to this journey. You've moved forward and toward your goals with each stride you've made, meal you've prepared, and ounce of commitment you've displayed.

Take with you the knowledge acquired, the tastes enjoyed, and the happiness derived from providing your body with healthful nourishment as you proceed beyond these pages. Recall that this is about a lifestyle change and a renewed understanding of the remarkable relationship between food and health, not just a diet.

Accept this experience's teachings and allow them to direct you as you proceed on your journey toward healing. Treat yourself with kindness, acknowledge and appreciate your successes, and see every day as a chance to make conscious, health-conscious decisions.

Now that you have this knowledge, these recipes, and this resolve, you can continue to thrive on this trip. Even if the road ahead may be twisted and turned, with the knowledge and skills you've acquired, you can handle it with poise and resiliency.

We appreciate you letting "Lose 30lbs in 30 Days" assist you with your change. Recall that this is only the start. One thoughtful decision at a time, your tale of health, energy, and success is beginning to take shape.

APPENDIX

METRIC CONVERSION CHART

Volume Conversions

- 1 teaspoon (tsp) = 5 milliliters (ml)

- 1 tablespoon (tbsp) = 15 milliliters (ml)

- 1 fluid ounce (fl oz) = 30 milliliters (ml)

- 1 cup = 240 milliliters (ml)

- 1 pint (pt) = 480 milliliters (ml)

- 1 quart (qt) = 0.95 liters (l)

- 1 gallon (gal) = 3.8 liters (l)

Weight Conversions (Dry Ingredients)

- 1 ounce (oz) = 28 grams (g)

- 1 pound (lb) = 454 grams (g)

- 1 kilogram (kg) = 1000 grams (g)

Temperature Conversions

- Celsius to Fahrenheit: $F = C \times 9/5 + 32$

  - 0°C = 32°F

  - 100°C = 212°F

- Fahrenheit to Celsius: $C = (F - 32) \times 5/9$

  - 32°F = 0°C

  - 212°F = 100°C

Length Conversions

- 1 inch (in) = 2.54 centimeters (cm)

- 1 foot (ft) = 30.48 centimeters (cm)

- 1 yard (yd) = 0.91 meters (m)

- 1 mile = 1.61 kilometers (km)

Oven Temperature Equivalents

- Low heat: 120°C - 150°C (250°F - 300°F)

- Moderate heat: 160°C - 180°C (325°F - 350°F)

- Moderate to high heat: 190°C - 230°C (375°F - 450°F)

- High heat: 240°C - 260°C (475°F - 500°F)

Common Kitchen Measurements

- 1 stick of butter = 113 grams (g) = 1/2 cup

- 1 liter of water = approximately 4 cups

- 1 kilogram of flour = approximately 8 cups

- 1 medium egg = approximately 50 grams (g)

Oven Racks Position

- Top rack: Generally for broiling or to brown the tops of dishes.

- Middle rack: For most baking and roasting.

- Bottom rack: Used for crisping crusts or cooking foods that require a lower temperature.

Liquid Measurements for Precision

- Use a liquid measuring cup for accurate volume measurements.

- Fill to the appropriate line by looking at the measurement at eye level.

INGREDIENT SUBSTITUITION GUIDE

In the journey towards healthier eating, flexibility in the kitchen can be your greatest ally. Understanding ingredient substitutions not only empowers you to adapt recipes to suit your dietary preferences but also allows for creative experimentation without compromising flavor or nutrition.

Here are some useful tips for ingredient substitution:

1. Sweeteners:

- **Natural Alternatives:** Replace refined sugars with healthier options like honey, maple syrup, or stevia for sweetness.

- **Fruit Purees:** Use mashed bananas or unsweetened applesauce in baking to reduce added sugars.

2. Fats:

-**Healthy Oils:** Opt for olive oil, avocado oil, or coconut oil instead of butter or margarine for a healthier fat profile.

- **Greek Yogurt:** Substitute part of the oil or butter in recipes with Greek yogurt for moisture and richness.

3. Flours and Grains:

- **Whole Grains:** Replace refined flours with whole wheat flour, almond flour, or oat flour for added fiber and nutrients.

- **Gluten-Free Options:** Experiment with gluten-free alternatives like rice flour, quinoa flour, or chickpea flour.

4. Dairy:

- **Plant-Based Milks:** Swap cow's milk with almond, soy, or oat milk for lactose-free and lower-calorie options.

- **Nutritional Yeast:** Use nutritional yeast as a cheesy substitute in recipes calling for cheese.

5. Proteins:

- **Plant-Based Proteins:** Incorporate tofu, tempeh, or legumes like beans and lentils as alternatives to meat for a lighter protein source.

- **Lean Meats:** Choose lean cuts of meat like skinless chicken or turkey for lower fat content.

6. Seasonings and Flavor Enhancers:

- **Herbs and Spices:** Experiment with fresh herbs and spices to add flavor without relying on excessive salt or seasoning blends.

Remember, while substitutions can often elevate the nutritional value of a dish, it's essential to consider the taste and texture changes that may occur. Feel free to tweak and adjust recipes to your liking, allowing your creativity to flourish in the kitchen while supporting your health and wellness goals.

Thank you

for embarking on this culinary journey. We hope these recipes have tantalized your taste buds and sparked joy in your kitchen.

*If you've enjoyed the flavors within these pages, **we kindly ask you to share your thoughts and experiences by KINDLY leaving a review.** Your feedback means the world to us and helps others discover the delights awaiting them in this cookbook.*

Happy cooking, and may your kitchen always be filled with laughter and delicious aromas!

www.ingramcontent.com/pod-product-compliance
Lightning Source LLC
Chambersburg PA
CBHW071608270726
48661CB00019B/1646